MY LIFE WITH TMJ DISORDER

BY

AILEEN RODRIGUEZ

This book is a work of non-fiction. Names and places have been changed to protect the privacy of all individuals. The events and situations are true.

ISBN: 1-4140-0052-9 (e-book)
ISBN: 1-4140-0051-0 (Paperback)

Library of Congress Control Number: 2003095274

This book is printed on acid free paper.

Printed in the United States of America
Bloomington, IN

1stBooks - rev. 08/05/03

The information in this book is
based on my personal experience with
TMJ Disorder.

It is not meant as a professional
approach. It is imperative to seek professional
advice and treatment.

CONTENTS

INTRODUCTION

After years of suffering from TMJ disorder, I noticed the lack of knowledge and information there was on the market about a disorder, which affects between 20 to 25 % of the population of the United States, its severity ranging from mild to severe. The majority of the cases, however, go untreated.

I also found so many professionals who were unaware of the symptoms of this disorder, mostly because in many cases the pain and discomfort is not specific in one area, but cover different parts of your body. From a tooth ache to backache or other areas which make it more difficult to diagnose and treat.

This book shares my experience and determination to find a solution and become the person I was before this disorder controlled every aspect of my life.

TMJ Disorder affects your jaw joints and its surroundings. But most of all, it affects you emotionally to the extent of becoming a person with low self esteem, feelings of depression, isolation, and at times, ill-tempered.

I would like to thank all those people in my life whom without them, I could not have finally found my life back.

My parents and aunt, who not only gave me moral support, but also helped with the expenses of the surgery. My three children, Amaris, Frances and Alexander for their patience and love through this ordeal.

A very special thanks to my loving husband, who was by my side every step of the way. Who supported all my decisions even, if at times he didn't totally agree with them.

Last but not least, our little pom, Amber, who kept watch days and nights, while I was recovering, and is still lying by my side as I am writing this book.

ONE

WHAT IS TMJ?

Temporomandibular joints are hinge joints that connect your cranium to your mandible. They are located right in front of your ears on each side of your head. The human skull has two main components: the cranium and the mandible. Two of the components of the cranium are the "Temporo", which means temporal bones, located on each side of the cranium close to the ears. The mandible is the U-shaped jawbone, which we use to chew our food. The mandible is the moving part of your skull. In order to move correctly, it must have healthy joints on each side connected to the cranium.

This very long and often mispronounced word is more commonly known as TMJ. In some cases you can find TMD when it is referred as a "Disorder" of your TMJ. In my book you would see it as TMJ Disorder. TMJ Disorder is when those joints and/or its surrounding tissues are not working properly.

During this chapter, I will explain some of the causes, symptoms, treatments and preventions. Please note that I am specifying some, because I am writing this book with the information I have acquired through my personal experience suffering from this disorder, and some research I have done in order to learn more about an ailment that was so unfamiliar, not only to me, as a patient, but to so many people I have had contact with through the years.

CAUSES
-   Daily wear and tear
-   Habits, such as chewing gum, grinding your teeth or clenching your jaw
-   Major trauma, such as an accident or a blow to the head or jaw
-   Various forms of arthritis
-   Weak joint structure

SYMPTOMS
-   Chewing causes pain
-   Jaw opening diminishes
-   Dull or aching pain in front of your ear or in your jaw muscle
-   Tenderness in your jaw muscle
-   Clicking or grinding sounds when you chew or open and close your mouth
-   Locking of the joint
-   Headaches, backaches, earaches or toothaches
-   Burning or tingling sensations inside your mouth, throat or inside your ear

- Tenderness and swelling on sides of your face
- Movement of the positioning of the jaw

TREATMENTS
- Mouth guard or splint: It helps reduce grinding your teeth or clenching your jaw. This could eventually help in reducing the pain and/or discomfort
- Physical Therapy: This may include exercises to stretch, strengthen and relax the muscles within the jaw joint area.
  There is also ultrasound therapy which helps in soothing the muscles and reduce inflammation.
- Anti-inflammatory medicines: These could be as simple as any over the counter pain medicines such as ibuprofen, or more complex treatments such as injections of a corticosteroid drug into your jaw muscle.
- Surgery: This should be the last resort, but if all else fails, this could be your only choice.

SURGERIES
- Disk Plication
- Arthroscopic surgery
- Orthognathic surgery
- Joint Reconstruction surgery
- Joint Replacement surgery
- Possibly other surgeries

POSSIBLE PREVENTIONS

- Avoid bad habits: Any form of activities which aggravate the joint. It could be as simple as chewing gum, chewing hard foods or opening and closing your mouth very widely.

  There may also be more complex ones as grinding your teeth or clenching your jaw. Which can be an unconscious action.

- Exercise: Find a form of exercise to relax your jaw muscles.

- Relax: Try to find some relaxing activity to avoid focusing your stress in your jaw area.

TWO

THE BEGINNING OF A LONG JOURNEY

As I turned 44 on May 29, 2002, I was approximately two months away from a surgery which was giving me the hope of finally seeing light at the end of the tunnel.

For thirty years, I had been feeling some type of TMJ discomfort. Yet, during the last ten years, the discomfort had developed into an active TMJ Disorder. For most of this time, I did not give it much thought. It was part of my daily life. Nothing had prepared me for the morning when I looked at myself in the mirror and saw a totally different person. From then on, my life became TMJ.

It all started as far back as my teenage years. I would wake up in the morning with soreness in my jaw area. I recall yawning several times, in order to make the discomfort disappear. So every time I felt the discomfort, I would just open and close my mouth several times and it was gone. I never mentioned this to anyone, because I honestly thought nothing of it.

As the years went by, I started working in a bank. By this time, I would feel it when I woke up, and during some stressful days at work. I would just open and close my mouth several times and everything was fine again. Again, I felt no need to tell anyone about this. However, the discomfort was becoming more frequent.

One September morning in 1991, I was driving my daughters to school, when I encountered a dump truck, who was collecting trash on the other side of the road. I noticed from afar that the truck was on the wrong side of the street. It was on the north side of the road, where cars travel west, yet it was facing east. I saw a car driving west about a block away, and noticed the truck driving to my lane, in order to avoid a collision with that car. As I saw this, I put the brakes on my car to avoid hitting the truck. The pavement was wet from a night of rain. Due to this, my car slid out of control and started spinning in circles. I recall screaming to my daughters to hold on. The last thing I remember was seeing the back end of the truck closing in on my windshield.

As soon as I opened my eyes, I jumped out of the car to check on my girls. They were standing away from the car, which made me realize that some time had elapsed. I must have lost consciousness for a very short time. My oldest daughter was complaining of pain around the area where she was wearing her seatbelt. Yet my youngest, was in more shock than anything else. Luckily, they both had been secured by seatbelt and a car seat.

As soon as the rescue arrived, they insisted I be taken to the hospital. I felt no pain, but they knew better. I had blood running down my forehead, from a wound on my head.

They asked me if I was wearing a seatbelt, to which I embarrassingly said no. That explained, the bruise on my forehead. As I looked at my dismantled car, I noticed the windshield. I had broken the windshield with my head! Years later, I found out this could have some connection to my TMJ.

By this time, my husband and aunt had arrived, and my husband told the rescue he would take me to the hospital. As soon as I got there, they took me inside and took some X-rays. They left me there for a few hours, and sent me home. It seemed it was a bad bruise, but I could recover at home.

I started feeling back pains, and neck pains due to the accident, so I started physical therapy for a few months. Nothing more was ever mentioned of my forehead, since I did not feel any pain after a few days and everything seemed to be without incident.

A year after the accident, I started hearing a clicking sound when I opened and closed my mouth. It only happened when I opened wide. So I just adjusted by not opening my mouth too wide. When I ate a sandwich or a burger, I would either open wide and hear the sound or press it down so I did not have to open as wide. It never occurred to me that this could be from the accident. After all, it was all in my head, because my mouth had not incurred any injuries.

One day as I was having a sandwich with a friend during our lunch break, I started hearing the clicking sound. I mentioned it to her, to which she even opened her mouth to show me she had clicking too. She told me she thought nothing of it, so I didn't either.

This clicking lasted for two or three years. I do not even know exactly when it actually stopped. One day I was eating a burger and realized I had no more clicking. I was so happy to be able to open my mouth without hearing a sound.

After a few months, I started feeling pain on both sides of my face, close to the ears. I started having massive headaches, which suddenly came to mind I had inherited those annoying headaches from my mother. The right side of my face was the one who I could say became intolerable.

I would wake up in the middle of the night with this excruciating pain. I would open and close my mouth, massage the sides of my face and my temples, hoping to find some relief. Sometimes it worked, but most of the time I had to take some over-the-counter pain medication. During the day, I would constantly be taking, Advil, Tylenol, Bayer, Motrin, anything I could lay my hands on, but the pain would not go away, would have temporary relief, but nothing else.

By this time, my mouth opening capabilities were starting to diminish. I was only able to get small portions of food in my mouth. I would cut foods in smaller pieces to feel comfortable. Yet, with such pain and inconvenience, I did nothing about it.

Once I recall, during a check up, complaining about the pain to my doctor. He mentioned that it could be related to stress. He asked if I had stress in my life. And I answered with a big YES!!! My doctor left it at that.

As long as I can remember, I have been a very stressed out person. Even as a young girl I felt stress in school. I always wanted things to be perfect. Then, as I became a woman and joined the work force, I did my job with great attention to detail. I was an over achiever and always thought I could do better. My life was full of self- created stress.

Yet at this specific time in my life, I was going through all kinds of stress. I had made a career in banking. Although I had graduated with a Bachelors Degree in Elementary Education, I enjoyed banking much more than I would have enjoyed a class full of students. That's what I thought when I was 22, a young professional woman with a very good job, making more money than what I would make as a beginning teacher.

Years passed and banking started changing its demands. But most of all I had changed. For years, although I always have loved my family above all else, my job had been my priority. Long hours outside the home and social demands were taking a toll on my family life. My oldest daughter, was a teenager, and needed me to be there, take her places and be more involved in her life. My two youngest were in elementary school and wanted their mom to be able to be a more active mom in school and at home. My husband wanted to have a wife who would sit and talk with him without the rush of everyday life. But most of all, I wanted to be there. I wanted to be present in my children's lives most of the time. I needed to take care of all their needs and not depend on my parents and aunt to care of those needs. I wanted to look back and tell them, how wonderful they did and not be told by someone else. In essence, I wanted my priority to be that of wife and mother and not my career.

This was not an easy thing to change. By this time I was making good money in banking, and changing implied a reduction in our financial situation. This took some planning. We started cutting all unnecessary things. We started focusing on the needs and not the wants. We paid our credit cards, and any outstanding debts. We had been fortunate to have bought our home when property values were extremely low. Therefore, we started paying off our mortgage.

It was not easy leaving my job, for a large group of students and a low paying teaching career. Getting used to a much smaller paycheck, and a different environment was hard to grasp. Yet, the first time I saw myself in front of a classroom, I realized all that I had missed. It was and still is a beautiful experience; to be able to make a difference in a child's life, and a difference in mine.

When the doctor related my problem to stress, I had no doubt he was right. I knew, after all these changes in my life, most of this annoying problem would ultimately go away. Little did I know, my problem was only going to get worse, to a point of total desperation.

I gradually started gaining some weight due to the stress. It was not a great deal, but I was fitting into size 10 pretty tightly and the evening dresses I had in my closet no longer fit right.

A few years passed, and my brother-in-law had set a date for his wedding. It was getting close to the wedding (exactly three weeks), and I could not afford to buy a new dress. I got into a very strict self made diet. I lost the weight I wanted and fit into one of my tightest dresses.

The day of the wedding, I was feeling sick. I could not explain what it was, but the feeling was not right. As soon as the wedding started, I had a need to use the bathroom. I went in and every time I had any intention of going out I had to go back and sit on the toilet. I was missing the entire wedding, and guests were starting to wonder where I was. When I finally finished, I looked inside the toilet and saw it filled with blood. I was very scared, but decided not to tell anyone in order not to ruin the celebration.

During the party, I had to excuse myself several times and every time I kept seeing great amount of blood. I had no choice but to tell my husband, and we left as soon as we could.

My husband insisted to go to the hospital, but I refused. I wanted to go home, take my clothes off and get comfortable. That's what we did. Before I went to bed, I went to the bathroom and there was less blood. So I figured it was getting better.

The following morning, as I was preparing breakfast, I felt something running down my legs. When I looked to see what it was, I saw a great deal of blood. This time I was so scared I told my husband we needed to go to the hospital. We left the kids at home, and left to the nearest hospital. I thought I was dying. I had never had rectal bleeding and never had seen this great amount of blood.

As soon as we arrived at the hospital, the nurse called me in. The doctor walked in a few minutes later, to which we explained what was happening. He explained that in order for him to know what was wrong, he had to do a colonoscopy. He explained the bright red blood, which was what I had been discharging, was a better sign than dark red. That made me feel better, but I kept worrying. He asked me to drink an ill-tasting liquid, which I reluctantly did.

I waited for an hour after I had finished the drink. I kept going to the bathroom over and over again. He wanted my intestines to be as empty as possible.

As I was being taken out of emergency to have the colonoscopy done, I looked at my husband and told him to take care of our children. I don't know why every time I am confronted with any situation, I think of them having to live life without me around to take care of them.

The procedure was a bit uncomfortable, yet painless. When I recovered, the doctor came in and said I had acute colitis.

I needed to know the reason a person would get acute colitis. He explained that this could be triggered by things I ate, or a stress filled lifestyle.

At that point I didn't put much thought into what I ate. It seemed I ate the same things other people ate. I didn't eat great amounts of junk foods. As a matter of fact, other than the couple of glasses of wine I drank every night and the cheese I ate while I was preparing dinner, everything else I ate was healthy.

Yet, I did pay attention to my "stress filled lifestyle". It didn't matter what I did I kept having stress. I no longer could blame it on my banking job and the long hours I put into it. Nor could I blame it on changing careers, and the financial cut backs we had. That was all in the past. Now, why was I still feeling stressed? The only thing I could think of was that I had to deal with the fact that I would find stress in every angle of my life. That was just the way I was. Either I let it control my life or I would have to start taking control of it. Easier said than done.

During my stay in the hospital, I was on a liquid diet and I.V. When I left the hospital I had shed a few more pounds and with no rectal bleeding.

The doctor gave me instructions to start eating pureed foods and take a week off from work. He mentioned to stop any extra activities I did for a while. My children and I taught catechism on Saturday mornings in our church, prepared Christmas plays and helped prepare the young children for their First Communion. I sadly had to stop that for a full year.

A week after I left the hospital, I started bleeding again. It wasn't as much as before, but I knew I had to call the doctor. Something was still wrong. As soon as I called the doctor, he requested I go to his office immediately. When I arrived, the nurse asked me to go in, and the doctor followed behind her. He looked at me and noticed my chest, hands and neck had a dark reddish appearance, and appeared to be swollen. The next thing I knew, he was referring me to an allergist. He thought my problem could be related to either food or environmental allergies.

When I got home, I called for an appointment. The following week, I went to see the allergist. It was a small and crowded office. For some reason it seemed children were more prone to allergies, since the office was full of small children. I waited there for a couple of hours, before they called me in. A young woman started the testing process. It seemed like an eternity, but I understood this needed to be very precise, and there were many things in the environment and different kinds of foods a person could be allergic to. She took notes as she was testing me. Then I went home, still not knowing what my allergies were.

The following week I went to see the allergist for the results of the tests. Indeed I was a very allergic person.

I had a number of environmental allergies, and more so, food allergies. Cherry, grape, celery, potato, bread, milk and any milk by product, such as cheese, butter, cream, yogurt etc. were all to be avoided. The hardest part of these allergies were that you did not know the ingredients that went into many products. I needed to read the ingredients carefully before buying anything. Even in restaurants, I had to ask what ingredients went into the meal I was ordering. She also put me on a shot therapy plan, which would last for approximately two years.

From this point on, I decided to start taking better care of myself. I made a menu plan, to make sure I did not eat any food I was not supposed to. Honestly, it was not very hard only for two things: the wine, I enjoyed drinking with my husband at night during dinner and the good old slices of cheese I loved to eat before dinner. Other than that, most of it was pretty easy, unless, mistakenly, I ate something not knowing what went into it.

Incredibly enough I lost the swelling, which I had not been aware of. As a consequence, I appeared much thinner.

Although I was not overweight before this, I enjoyed being called slim. Yet the best thing was I had no more rectal bleeding.

Due to the sudden weight loss, the skin around my lips started sagging. I had heard of an over the counter device that you put inside your mouth and exercise, in order to get some muscle back in the area. I ordered one and started using it. I did the exercises three times a day every single day for a month or so. I did notice an improvement in the toning of the muscle around my lips, so my plan was to keep using this miracle device.

Suddenly, one morning as I was getting ready for work, I was putting my makeup on, when I noticed a dramatic change in my facial anatomy.

I could not believe what I was seeing in that mirror. Nothing could have prepared me for this. My face seemed to have shifted to the left. The right side of my face had thinned out, while the left seemed plump. As I looked closer, I noticed that my chin had protruded. I had developed an asymmetrical face. As far as I was concerned, this was a facial deformity. I didn't know if this had happened suddenly overnight or if this was something that had slowly progressed. Maybe the sagging around my lips was a sign of the beginning of this facial change, and not the weight I had lost. Whatever the reason, I was feeling devastated.

My facial anatomy prior to this was squared jaw line, of which nothing was left of it. I never considered myself a very beautiful woman, but more than anything somewhat attractive. There was nothing left of that now.

This day changed my life forever. I knew then I was going to get to the root of this.

At the beginning, I could not talk about it to anyone, because I was still convinced it was a bad dream. All the aches and pains I was suffering were nothing compared to this. The mirror became an obsession. I would go to the bathroom during my classroom breaks, just to look at myself in the mirror, hoping this would change. Yet, I kept looking the same.

I knew people noticed, but didn't dare say anything. Some people would say I was losing too much weight. Others would ask if I was sick. But the worse pain came from my oldest daughter. She was born when I was 19, and I was the youngest mom in her group of friends. She would always tell me how pretty I was. Her compliments were present all the time. Although I didn't pay much attention to them then, all of a sudden the lack of compliments tortured me.

I finally decided to tell someone. Whom better than my husband, who was so close to me and had the tendency of being extremely honest. This time I needed honesty. I asked him to look at my face and tell me what he saw. Did he notice any changes? At first he said I looked the same as always. Then I started to cry, because I knew he was trying to make me feel good.

I have always been very self-conscience about my looks. I never left the house looking anything less than what I considered perfect. My husband knew that. We had been together for years, and he knew that was a very delicate subject with me.

I insisted and he agreed that my face had changed dramatically. His honesty hurt, but was much appreciated. He even told me I needed to find out the cause of this change.

Talking about it with him, helped me realize I needed to seek professional help. The sooner the better.

Who would I turn to?

THREE

GOING ROUND IN CIRCLES

Having heard the truth from my husband convinced me this was actually real. If I needed help I had to start talking about it and asking many questions.

It took me several weeks to be able to talk to my family about it, but they had to know. I told my parents and my aunt what I was going through. Indeed they had noticed, but had decided not to mention it to me. They knew it was not life threatening, but were afraid of how I would feel if they told me they had noticed.

By this time, I had developed a very low self-esteem. I was afraid to see old friends from high school or from work. Those people I had not seen in years, were the ones I feared to see most. It was coming to a point, where I just wanted to do my daily routines and not participate in any social events. The love of my family and my sense of responsibility kept me away from falling into a deep depression. If it weren't for that, I would have laid in bed for days and not go out of the house.

Internally, I felt like an old woman. The aches and pains would not go away. As a matter of fact, they were getting worse as each day passed. My allergies were controlled due to a strict diet. Yet, if I ate anything to which I was allergic, not only would I swell, but if it was bad enough I would have some rectal bleeding.

There was so much going on inside of me, yet I didn't associate one illness with the other. I felt each was a separate entity.

For several weeks I kept asking around and no one seemed to know. One day my aunt suggested I see a neurologist. I had doubts, since in my opinion a neurologist treats the brain. Yet in researching, my aunt was right. This specialist diagnoses and treats diseases of the nervous system, and this could be a possibility. So I decided to look for a good one.

I went into a comfortable office full of patients. I thought I would have to wait, but after filling out the insurance forms I was called in immediately.

The doctor walked in and asked me to explain what I was feeling. I limited myself to telling him about my facial change to which I asked if it could be related to a disease of my nervous system. He examined me. Then he asked if I was feeling any pains, to which I started telling him about the headaches and pain in front of my ears and some neck and back pain. I did not let him say a word, and immediately told him I thought it was all related to stress. The doctor agreed it could be, yet told me I had no neurological problems, and should be treated based on those pains. He did notice my teeth were not aligned and told me to seek the assistance of a dentist. This lack of information, caused me to become anxious and somewhat more depressed about my ailment.

The following day, I gave my dentist a call. I had little faith he could do anything about it, but I needed to keep trying. He gave me an appointment for the following week.

I entered his small and crowded office, thinking again of the wait. Yes, I did have to wait a very long time. As a matter of fact, I was the last patient to be seen. I sat in the dental chair and waited some time before the dentist came in. Again, I was asked the same question, and again began telling my story. This time I started with the facial changes, but then I continued with all the aches and pains. I could not forget the teeth alignment, that was the reason the neurologist said I should see my dentist in the first place.

He started examining me. He asked me to open my mouth as wide as I could. He kept insisting that I open wider. I tried, but could not open anymore than I was doing. He gave me a mirror so that I could see where my teeth touched when I closed my mouth. The bottom teeth were shifted to the left. In short, they were not centered. He said this could be corrected orthodontically. Then he mentioned the openning of my mouth, and said I should be able to open wider. For that he recommended a periodontist, who worked inside the same office.

When I left my dentist's office, I had the appointment to see the periodontist. It was two months away.

I decided I would wait to see the orthodontist until I had seen the periodontist. I already had braces as an adult and was not very excited about getting them again.

For two months I waited, hoping this doctor would shed some light on the subject. I tried keeping myself busy, to avoid thinking much about my situation, but to no avail. During this time my level of pain became worse. Sometimes, I would wake up crying in the middle of the night, because of the terrible pain I was having. Through all this time, I thought the acute pain was a result of my state of mind.

For the first time in all these years, I started wondering if the pain and the facial changes would possibly be related.

Finally, the much anticipated day came. I sat in his office, and prayed that he could find a reason for my situation. I needed to know what was happening to my body and could not wait any longer.

I heard the young woman call my name, and as I walked in, the doctor greeted me. He took me to his office and examined me. He seemed to know my story, since my dentist worked in the same office, and he was reading my file. He asked me to open and close, then asked me to close my mouth and put my teeth together. While I had my mouth closed, he touched the front of my ear. In the slightest touch, I felt great pain. While leaving his fingers in that position, he asked me to open and close my mouth, several times.

Upon finishing with this exam, he explained my problem. My mandible or lower jaw had shifted due to some problem in my joint. That was the reason for my facial change, the pain I was feeling in front of my ears and my teeth alignment condition. Then came what I hoped I would not hear. He could not treat my condition. This called for an Oral and Maxillofacial Surgeon.

I desperately needed a name and a good recommendation of an oral and maxillofacial surgeon. Fortunate for me, the periodontist knew one he considered the best in our area. I got the name and the telephone number from his assistant before leaving his office.

That night, as I left the doctors office, I felt a sense of relief. He had provided me with more information than anyone I had seen before. Now I knew what my problem was. All I needed now was to go to the doctor who could cure me.

I had no choice but to wait until Monday. Monday morning, bright and early I was calling the oral and maxillofacial surgeon. The receptionist answered and gave me an appointment in two months. I could not believe this doctor did not have any availability through the remaining of the summer. Here I was during summer break, hoping to treat my condition and the only doctor who could do that gave me the appointment for the end of September. I figured, I had to accept it. I was a new patient and had to wait as long as I had to.

FOUR

THE JOURNEY GOES ON

It was a Monday afternoon in late September, when I walked into a small and very crowded office. I went in, wrote my name on the sign in sheet and stood against a wall waiting for someone to be called in so I could sit down.

It had been an exhausting day with the students. I hadn't had a chance to eat lunch and at dismissal it was pouring rain. This meant, waiting in the school cafeteria, until all the children had been picked up. What had kept me going in such a positive mood was the afternoon appointment I was going to have.

While I was waiting, I started analyzing the faces around me. I was hoping to see an assymetrical face like mine to make sure I was in the right place. Yet I saw none. Finally a gentleman is called in and I could sit and relax. I began a conversation with the lady sitting next to me. I asked why she was there, and she told me she was waiting for her son who was having a wisdom tooth extracted. At first I thought there was another doctor working with the oral and maxillofacial surgeon, because I thought only

28

regular dentists did this. I asked the lady if the oral and maxillofacial surgeon was extracting the tooth and she said yes. Then she explained that the dentist was not able to extract the wisdom tooth due to complications and sent her son to this doctor.

I waited for so long, I even fell asleep for a while. The sound of my name woke me up. It was his assistant calling me in. She took me for X-rays. These were not the average X-rays, they produce a panoramic image of the jaw from ear to ear.

The first X-ray was taken standing up facing the machine. A part of the machine would turn around circling my head. The second one was taken as I was sitting down. Two small pieces were slightly pressed into my ear and a side X-ray was taken. I waited for a few moments to make sure they did not have to be retaken, then she took me into an examining room. I sat down in the dental chair and waited for the doctor to come in.

A few minutes later, the doctor walked in. After introducing himself, he asked me the same question I had been asked so many times before. I explained to him all the pains I was feeling for years. How it would wake me up in the middle of the night, all the massages I would do to alleviate the pain, and all the pain medication I was taking on a daily basis. Then I started talking to him about my primary concern, my face. Would I ever look the same again?

He examined me without saying a word. He asked me to open and close my mouth several times. He asked me to open as wide as I could, then close again and have my teeth from my upper and lower jaw touch. He touched my head, especially the part around my ears. He pressed his finger on the top and back part of my ear as well as the front. Every place he touched I felt a great deal of pain. As a matter of fact, I felt greater pain on the right side. He asked me to move my bottom jaw from side to side and toward the front. I could barely do that. It was as if my jaw was locked. His assistant came in with the X-rays so he could see them. He took a few moments from the examination in order to carefully look at them.

He gave me a mirror so I could see myself as he gave me an explanation. He asked me to open my mouth and showed me how I was not opening straight. This was due to the inferior border of the left mandible that was higher than the right. Opening was very limited, between 30-35 mm.

Then he asked me to close my mouth and open my lips so I could look at my teeth. Only some teeth were touching, and explained I had an open bite, where only the left posterior molars were in contact with each other. There was wear on the top part of my teeth indicating I would grind my teeth or clench my jaw. Again he showed me my teeth, where he pointed that the midline had shifted. I then moved my jaw sideways, where he showed me the limitation I had by demonstrating himself. The last thing he showed me was as I moved my jaw forward. It was moving to one side and not straight as it should.

After these demonstrations, he explained what he saw in the X-rays. The panorex studies showed osteoarthrosis of the left mandibular condyle. The right seemed to maintain a seminormal projection. Then he explained I needed more testings in order to give me a complete diagnosis of my condition. All this explained my facial assymetry. But did not explain why my right side was in more pain than my left. I would have to wait to find out.

He wanted me to be aware of any pressure I would put on my jaw. He explained to me that many people release their stress either by grinding their teeth or clenching their jaw. Most of the time, people are not aware they are doing it. It can also happen as they sleep. He explained this disorder I was having was called TMJ disorder, and it affected more women than man, mostly because its more likely that a woman releases her stress by placing pressure in that area. I repeated those three letters, yet did not think to ask what the acronym stood for. I only thought of those letters causing in me such a big problem.

Before I left his office, he gave me a treatment plan and more precise testings:

- Soft Diet- This was basically a non-chew diet.
- M.R.I. -This is short for Magnetic Resonance Imaging.
- Therapy- This was requested so I could learn how to relax my jaw.
- Orthodontist- This request was for making a splint, which I would wear mostly at night, but I could use it anytime I felt stress around my jaw area. Also, for examination for possible orthognathic correction (I would mention this more specifically in coming chapters).

He wanted to see me in twelve weeks, so he could check on my progress, especially the therapy and the splint.

I left his office with mixed emotions. I was very happy I found the right doctor, who could treat me. His diagnosis made great sense to me, which answered so many questions. On the other hand, I was concerned about the ultimate cure, if any. It seemed, I was in worse shape than I had anticipated.

The following day I made the appointments for the M.R.I., therapist and orthodontist. Within a week, I had been to all three. I went to the hospital for the M.R.I. This was a scary sight, since it was a closed M.R.I. and you lie down, they pushed you into a long tube, where you barely fit and then they do the testing which lasted approximately 45 minutes. The therapist on the other hand was a very relaxing experience. Not only did I learn certain techniques to relax my jaw area, but I also learned how to relax other parts of my body as well. I would have to go to therapy 3 times a week for 12 weeks. I visited the orthodontist, where they took models of my teeth and a week later, they gave me the splint.

Twelve weeks later, I was back at the doctor's office. Again, the office was very crowded. So full that patients were waiting outside sitting on some benches across from the elevators.

I was called in about an hour later. I was taken to the examining room, where the assistant placed the copies of the M.R.I., already examined by the doctor. As he walked in, he was nodding his head. He was concerned about the time I had waited to seek help. He asked me to open and close my mouth as wide as I could, which I did with much limitation. He was trying to hear a clicking sound, but there was none. I explained to him I had clicking in my jaw years earlier, but it had suddenly stopped. It had been years since I heard the clicking, which I assumed it meant that whatever I had there must have been cured.

The doctor left the office to find the model of a skull. The model showed a perfect jaw joint with perfect movement. He explained through the model the different parts of the TMJ or Temporomandibular Joint. He pointed at the temporal bone, which is part of the cranium. Under that there is an enlarged and rounded bone called a condyle. The condyle is part of the mandible, which is the moving part. Between the temporal bone and the condlye there is a softer tissue whose function is to lubricate the joint in order to facilitate the movement and avoid the bones rubbing against each other. This is called cartilage, which we have in all areas of our body, which have joints. In addition, the TMJ has a special fibrous cartilage which makes it more flexible and its called articular disk. When in the opening and closing of the mouth the articular disk escapes the condyle, then clicking may occur. Sometimes the clicking goes away, because the disk no longer escapes the condyle. But in the worse case scenario, the clicking would go away due to the articular disks moving away from its correct place and the temporal bones and the condyles would rub against each other. As a result of this, the bones degenerate. When there is bone degeneration there is pain associated with it, the jaw opening would be reduced, normal chewing would be impossible, speech could be affected and jaw movement occurs.

After the doctor finished his explanation, I knew my case was the latter one. It showed all of my symptoms, except for speech impediment.

During the three months prior to this visit, I had been concentrating on everything I did with my jaw. I even woke up in the middle of the night, with a clenched jaw. I was so focused on my jaw that I realized, I clenched at different times during the day. That explained the soreness I had in my jaw area for so many years. Now I was conscious of what I was doing, and I was going through therapy, I knew that when I started clenching I could relax my jaw by doing my relaxation exercises. During the night, I would wear the splint and I would not clench my jaw. The pain had diminished a bit. I was not taking as many pain medications as I had prior to these three months. Yet I had two main concerns: How could I avoid more degeneration of my condyles?, and How could I get my face the way it was before all this happened?

The doctor had no answers for me at that time. As a matter of fact, he had more questions than answers himself. He wanted to do an arthroscopic surgery of the right temporomandibular joint. This is performed with the assistance of an arthroscope, which is a miniature microscope in order to look into the joint. A small puncture through the skin is done to introduce the arthroscope, get a biopsy and wash area with a salt-water solution in order to open up the joint space, and relief some of the pain.

He gave me the appointment for the arthroscopic surgery for Friday of the following week.

FIVE

SURGERY NUMBER 1

Friday morning I arrived at his office. I had nothing to eat or drink since midnight. I have to admit, I was a bit nervous, since I knew I would be awake through this although minor, but uncomfortable surgery.

At 8:30 his assistant called me in to the surgery room. She placed a cap on my head and covered me with a warm blanket. The doctor walked in a few minutes later, and showed me the arthroscope he would use for this surgery. He also asked me to lie on my left side, so he could work on the right. He showed a small screen where he would be looking at the joint in a magnified way. He suggested I could look at the screen so I could see what was happening. Before he started, he explained that he was working on the right side rather than the left, because the pain level on the right was greater than on the left. Also, the right side was less degenerated and could benefit more from this procedure.

He administered various shots to numb the area. Then he introduced the arthroscope and began observing at the screen, examining the area of the joint. As he examined the joint, he explained what he was looking at. But in all honesty, I was afraid to look, and was so nervous I was not listening to a word he said. He took a biopsy of the joint, he manipulated the articular disk gently and he put the water solution to increase motion and alleviate pain.

Then he took the arthroscope out and closed my skin with two stitches. I remained there for a few minutes, then was taken to another room, where my parents were waiting. As soon as the doctor noticed I was feeling better, he released me.

I went home and rested the entire weekend. On Monday morning, I was back at work. I was swollen and had the two stitches, but other than that I felt good. The following Friday, I went to his office to have the stitches removed by his assistant.

I would continue therapy for three more months, would wear the splint at night and would remain on a soft diet.

I was starting to feel better. The pain level on my right joint had diminished about 50%. I could feel I was opening my mouth more, with less discomfort. It all seemed to be improving.

Three months later I visited the doctor. I felt much better, as far as the pain and discomfort were concerned. They did more x-rays, which showed my joints were stable. In other words, no more degeneration had ocurred. This was a good sign, because if the joints were stable, the doctor would consider an alternative surgery to correct my jaw, and this would fix my facial deformity.

The doctor wanted to see me in three more months. At this time, he would consider whether orthonagnathic surgery would be a good alternative for my jaw correction.

As I started learning more about my condition, I realized that my doctor was trying to avoid going into the joint due to complications which may arise. When the doctor mentioned his decision to have my facial asymmetry corrected with orthognathic surgery, I considered it to be the best choice for me.

Orthognathic surgery is nothing else than jaw-correcting surgery. Notice I didn't say joint - correcting, and that is because the joint, though it's defective in my case, will not be worked on.

Three months went by and I was back in the doctor's office. Again, his assistant took some x-rays. As soon as the doctor saw them, he told me we had good news. The joints on both sides had maintained their stability since my last visit. This gave him confidence that orthognathic surgery was my best choice.

He explained this surgery had no guarantees, due to the joint's stability. If the joint continued to degenerate in the future, my jaw would move again and the operation would have failed. I heard all this, but had faith that my joint had already degenerated all that it was going to degenerate. For months, I had been taking all sorts of vitamins to regenerate my joints. With all that and all I had learned about joint relaxation, I was hopeful this would be a permanent solution.

I was glad to hear this, because I now had the hope of having my facial deformity corrected. I could be myself again.

I hoped to soon look at myself in the mirror and be happy with what I saw. I could face my old friends and be the person I was before this nightmare started.

This was not going to happen any time soon. The doctor explained that he had to submit all the paperwork to the insurance, because some insurances were not paying for this surgery. Then, if it was approved I would have to go back to the orthodontist and have braces put on.

The braces had to be on for at least six months prior to surgery. The orthodontist would try to correct my bite in a way that my teeth would fall into place when the jaw was corrrected.

I waited for six weeks, before I got a call from the doctor's office saying that the insurance had approved my surgery. So I called the orthodontist for an appointment to have my braces put on.

On July 2000, I got braces. Then every four weeks I would go to have them adjusted. During this time, the orthodontist kept close contact with my doctor in order to monitor my progress. I visited the doctor for follow up during this time. This process lasted one whole year. Quite a bit more than we had anticipated.

Finally, the day arrived when the orthodontist gave me the green light. I visited my doctor the following week and we scheduled the surgery in six weeks. It could not be any earlier, because I needed to go to the Red Cross to donate 2 pints of blood for the surgery. This was done in 2 week intervals. Also, I was put on a high iron diet and vitamins for six weeks. During this visit, his assistant gave me some legal forms to initial. All that I initialed I had previously been informed, yet I wanted to read it to refresh my memory.

Basically the risks were as follows:
- Damage to the infraorbital nerve either temporary or permanent.
- Problems developing in the sinus.
- Damage to the teeth or roots of teeth, which could result in extraction or endodontic procedure.
- Loss of bone secondary to infection or lack of blood supply.
- Non-union, mal-union or relapse requiring more surgery.
- Comprise of nasal airways (post surgery)

Honestly, I never thought any of the above mentioned would happen to me. All that came into my mind was that I was going to have my face back to the way it was. And that was enough for me.

The doctor explained with the same model of a skull he had previously used, where he was going to cut the bone on both sides of the mandible. Then he would put two metal plates with screws to straighten my jaw. Also, he was going to extract a wisdom tooth that could create a problem after the surgery. The great thing about this surgery was that it was all going to be done inside the mouth, so I would not have any noticeable scars.

The surgery was scheduled for July 17, 2001.

SIX

SURGERY NUMBER 2

The day prior to my surgery, I went to the hospital for my pre-op. That day I signed some paperwork for the insurance and they did some lab test on me. The following day was the big day. I could have nothing to eat or drink after midnight.

It was 5:00 A.M. when my husband and I woke up. My three children would stay home until the surgery was over and they would go to see me. I have to admit I was not as nervous as I was on the first surgery. It could have been the joy I was feeling inside of me, that after a few hours I could look at myself in the mirror and see a totally new person, or rather the person I had been.

We arrived in the hospital at 6:00 A.M. They called me in, prepared me for the surgery, I.V. and all. I waited approximately an hour for the anesthesiologist to come in. She explained I would be sleeping through general anesthesia via nasotracheal intubation. By 8:00 they took me into the operating room. I was very happy to see those so familiar faces, my doctor and his assistant. I looked straight at my doctor and told him to make me pretty again. All I can remember was him smiling at my comment. When I woke up, the first thing I asked was if I looked pretty.

Funny I asked such question, because as soon as I got a room after recovery, I insisted that my husband would bring me a mirror so I could take a good look at myself.

It was not a pretty sight. All I could see was my head and most of my face covered with gauze. The small part of my face I could see was so swollen it did not look like me at all.

My husband told me the swelling would last for a while, but the doctor had said the surgery had gone extremely well.

The day after the surgery, I was released from the hospital. The doctor wanted me to go to his office for a panorex x-ray. The doctor's office connects to the hospital, so I sat in a wheel chair and the nurse took me there. As soon as I arrived, his assistant took a panorex, which the doctor saw and told me it showed good anatomical position of the plates and screws. The condyles had remained stable during the surgery, which was a very good sign.

I felt numbness on the left side of my face and on the bottom lip, but that was expected. The numbness should go away after six months, but there are some cases where some numbness could be permanent.

I had a splint pressed together by heavy elastics. This would keep my mouth immobile. The elastics would be the most important part of the recovery. The doctor showed me how to take them off to eat (basically liquid or pureed foods), and brush my teeth, then I must put them back on. This would remain like this until he dictated otherwise. When I left his office, I was on antibiotic and pain medication.

I was in bed for the whole week. The excruciating pain I was having made me wonder if this was normal for this kind of surgery. My husband kept insisting to call the doctor, but like most things in my life, I resisted hoping it would be getting better. The pain medication would alleviate the pain for a while, then it would start again.

Between the pain and the liquid diet, which I was resisting to eat made me so weak, I could barely stand up.

Incredibly enough, the pain was not in the bone of my mandible, it was in my palate, inner cheek and inner lip. Also, the left side of my face was as swollen as the first day of the surgery, yet the right side, which was where the pain was, started showing signs of unswelling.

A week and a half after the surgery I returned to the doctor's office. I was feeling so weak, I was practically dragging my feet. My aunt drove me to the doctor's office, and I literally had to hold on to her, an already elderly woman with problems walking herself.

As soon as they saw me, the assistant immediately took me in and lay me down on the bed, where the doctor had conducted the arthroscopic surgery. The doctor came in and took off the splint and elastics so I could explain what was happening to me. He examined inside my mouth where I was claiming so much pain, and he noticed the wiring and the splint were scratching those areas. He then removed the drainage I had on the surgery site, and checked the healing on both sides of my mandible. The right side was healing properly, but the left side had a yellowish sanguinous discharge. This did not look good. The discharge meant there was some kind of infection.

He decided to leave the splint out and place the heavy elastics wrapped in the surgical hooks I had on my braces. He put me on a stronger antibiotic, and told me to go home and get some food in my body. He wanted to see me the following day. When I left his office, I was feeling much better. That excruciating pain was gone and I was feeling up to having something to eat.

When I got home, my mother was waiting with some black bean soup for dinner. The lack of pain and that black bean soup made a big difference in the way I was feeling. I even sat on the couch with my kids to watch some T.V. That was a first since the surgery.

The following day, I returned to the doctor's office. Everyone noticed how much better I looked from the previous day. The doctor was very happy to see the change in my appearance, to which he mentioned, I had him scared the day before. Then he took the elastics and concentrated on the left side. He explained that the wound was not healing due to an infection. I still had the discharge, which was a concern for him as well as for me. He gave me a syringe, so I could fill with warm water and salt to cleanse the wound. He kept me on the same antibiotic he prescribed the day before. He wanted to see me in 10 days.

I left his office ready to do whatever it took to get that wound healed. So I cleansed three times a day, kept taking the antibiotic and tried eating as healthy as I could.

Instead of improving, I was feeling weaker as each day passed. This time I would have called my doctor, but I knew he was out of town. I'm sure someone would have tried to help me if I would have called, but I thought if it got really bad I would just go to the hospital.

When I returned to his office, the swelling had not gotten any better. I was feeling so weak, I did not care anymore what I looked like. I just wanted to feel better.

He checked the left side and the discharge was still there causing the wound to remain open. He then changed me to a different antibiotic. On this visit a new problem arose, tooth #18 was mobile. This was caused by the infection.

A panorex x-ray was taken which looked quite good. No problem was seen on the x-ray as to a loose screw, movement of bone plate or slippage of the fracture site. Though the widening of the periodontal ligament on tooth #18 was noticed. He wanted to see me in 72 hours.

During this time, I was feeling weaker and weaker. I would spend most of the day in bed, watching T.V., not wanting to eat or get up to just look out a window. On the third day, I returned to his office. He immediately noticed the weakness, and showed true signs of concerns for my well-being. Having run out of options to cure my infection, he called an infectious disease specialist to discuss my situation. He wanted to attempt one last time on by mouth antibiotic therapy, before thinking of other options. The infectious disease specialist suggested he prescribed a very potent antibiotic. He did specify I could feel weaker, because of the potency of this antibiotic, but it was his last resort. If this one did not work, I would have to go back to the operating room.

The next few days, were the worst I had felt since the surgery. I spent all the time in bed, feeling to weak to even go to the bathroom, and only was capable of drinking fruit juices. Everything else made me nauseous.

After six days, I went to his office one last time. Realizing my condition was worsening and my body was weakening, he decided the wound had to be re-opened, cleansed and checked, possibly removing the metal plate on the left side and extracting tooth #18.

Six weeks after the surgery, I was ready to go back to the operating room. This time, my concern was in curing my infection, so I could feel better. The last thing I had in my mind was how I looked. For the first time, since I have had TMJ disorder, I was concerned about my inner health rather than my outer appearance. This taught me where my priorities should be and not where they were.

My doctor would not be alone during this surgery. He would be working with the infectious disease specialist to determine what course of action would be taken after the surgery to rid my body or this infection. My doctor had warned me once those doctors were called in they would use the most aggressive therapy to cure the patient. This meant a very probable consideration of a long-term I.V antibiotic therapy.

I was devastated, but I knew there was no other choice. This situation needed to be remediated at once before it weakened my body anymore.

I needed to feel better for myself and most of all for my family. During those six weeks, they took care of all my needs. I needed to take charge and care for my needs, and mostly care for theirs. This had to be resolved.

The surgery was scheduled for the following day, September 6, 2001.

SEVEN

SURGERY NUMBER 3

The surgery was scheduled for noon. I arrived at 9:00 A.M., exactly one hour before I was called in. In the hospital lobby, close to the nurses station, there was a scale. I got up to weigh myself. I had lost approximately 20 pounds. Incredibly all my obsessions, including being thin were no longer as important as they were before. My main priority was to be healthy.

When I was called in, the nurse prepared me for the surgery. The anastheseologist walked in and explained the type of anesthesia he was using. It was exactly the same one I had on the previous surgery, only six weeks before.

This time I was really scared. I was very aware things can and do go wrong.

During the surgery, the doctor opened the wound, explored and cleaned it. He removed the metal plate, since the screws were so loose one of them popped out as he opened the wound. The jaw bone had regenerated and the removal of the plate would not affect the position of my jaw. He did not extract tooth #18, because he had hopes of saving it. This time a drainage was placed in the wound with heavy gauze.

As I woke from the surgery, a very strange feeling was taking place inside my body. It seemed as if my inner body wanted to explode. I couldn't explain it to the nurse, because my mouth was shut with heavy elastics. She proceeded to give me some pain medication, and after a few minutes it all went away.

The day after my surgery, the infectious disease physician came in to see me. After intruducing himself, he started explaining to me why my doctor had called him in. I had acquired a bone infection, which was difficult to say how I got it, but it had to be cured. For the past several weeks I was given many by mouth antibiotics and they did not cure the infection. This time, it was necessary to have the antibiotic going directly into my blood stream. In order to do this, I would need to have a PIC line opened for six weeks so I could administer the antibiotic directly into my blood. I was not thrilled with this option, but I accepted it.

A few minutes later, I was taken to have the PIC line placed. The doctor put some local anesthesia, and explained that a PIC line was nothing more than a fancy I.V. The Pic line was introduced on my left, upper arm. The line was then pushed in through my vein to reach my heart. Approximately 18 inches of line were left outside my body for my convenience as I would administer the antibiotic.

When I left the hospital that afternoon, I went to the infectious disease office. There I met the pharmacist and nurse who would help me through this. First, the nurse changed the bandages they placed in the hospital, cleaned the area around the line, placed new bandages and drew blood from the line. Then she proceeded to show me how to administer the antibiotic. It was a process that lasted about one hour. The good thing was I could be administering the antibiotic and doing other things at the same time. Then the pharmacist came in with a white cooler full of all the supplies I needed for a whole week. The syringes, alcohol, gauze and the antibiotics, which had to remain in a cool place at all times. Only the one I would use within the next eight hours would remain at room temperature. This would be a weekly visit to clean and draw blood and get the week's supply.

When I got home that night, I realized I was on my own. I had no doctors or nurses to help me clean and introduce the antibiotic into the line. I looked at my husband and my parents, who were reluctant to leave until they saw how I could get the antibiotic in. I was so afraid to do it myself, so I asked someone to help me. They appeared more scared than me. I knew it was not fair for me to ask anyone to do it for me, I had to be strong and learn. I started reading the instructions the nurse had written down, and started cleaning the line, connecting the antibiotic to the line, leaving it there for about 45 minutes, then cleaning the line one last time and closing it. Then I rolled the outside line into a net like arm brace the nurse had given me to avoid pulling the line.

It was a great relief when I finally finished. I knew the first time would be the hardest and would be getting better with time.

During the weekend, I started feeling symptoms of depression. I could not pin-point the cause. Was it the surgery or the PIC Line? I felt like a prisoner inside my own home. Although I was feeling stronger and was sure this was going to ultimately make me feel better, it was a feeling of despair I could not explain.

The following Monday, I visited my doctor where he removed the drainage. That was enough for me to break out in tears. I guess that was what I needed to release everything I had inside, because after I left his office I felt much better.

As the days went by, the swelling on the left side of my face was diminishing, and tooth #18 was getting stronger. That was great news, because this meant the infection was beginning to subside. This time I was so focused on the left side that I had not realized my face was beginning to look symmetrical. My oldest daughter brought this to my attention one day when she said I was starting to have the same face I had before. My daughter's comment meant a lot to me. I went straight to a mirror to look at my face and what I saw was to me some kind of miracle. My true facial expression was coming back. This, emotionally made me feel much better. Yes, I did have the inconvenience of the PIC line, but this was exactly what I needed to feel and look better.

My daughter was getting married in three months, and her bridal shower was taking place in the end of October.

As it was getting closer to the shower, I started itching all over and getting rashes in different parts of my body. Like what I had always done, I blamed it on stress. Preparing a big wedding and the shower was more than my nerves could handle at this specific time. Then it clicked, blaming everything on stress was what had gotten me in trouble in the first place. I immediately called my doctor.

He told me to call the infectious disease physician to tell him my problem.

The doctor told me to go to his office at once. I showed him the rash and explained the itching all around my body, then he concluded I had developed an allergic reaction to the antibiotic. He changed me to a different kind of antibiotic and gave me a week's supply of the new one.

I went home that afternoon and started on my new antibiotic. That night I was unable to sleep with all the itching. The rash was spreading to the rest of my body, so I called him early in the morning. He wanted to see me immediately. I got dressed and was in his office in no time.

He looked at me and concluded my body was saturated. He had estimated six weeks and I was already on my fifth, so he decided to remove the line and put me on by mouth antibiotic for two more weeks.

The day of my daughter's bridal shower I felt like a new person. Everyone was complimenting me on my looks. One family member said I looked like my old self only thinner.

I can't lie, it felt great to hear those words. Yet, after going through all this ordeal, those words were not what I longed for anymore.

I felt healthy and strong, had a beautiful family who had stood by me. My daughter was about to get married to a wonderful man. Nothing could feel better than that.

Yes, I felt attractive, but most of all I felt thankful to God for giving me the opportunity to see life in a different perspective.

For six more months, I would continue on a soft non-chew diet, wearing braces and elastics to rearrange my teeth.

EIGHT

ANOTHER JOURNEY BEGINS

Towards the end of November, I went to my orthodontist for my monthly visit. As he examined, he was surprised, as I was developing an open bite again. He called my doctor, which he immediately requested to see me.

As he examined me, he did notice a small open bite, but did not seem concerned at the time. He explained that when the jaw bones are broken as mine were, it temporarily stops blood flow to the joint and some slight changes could occur. I explained to him that I was starting to feel some pain in my joint and headaches which didn't seem to improve with the relaxation exercises. He suggested I take some anti-inflammatory over the counter medication.

That night before I went to bed, I analyzed my face in the mirror and noticed a slight change in my facial anatomy. This time I was convinced I would not think about it too much, and focus on the more positive aspects of my life.

The day my daughter got married was a very stressful day. I hardly slept the night before, thinking of all the things we had to do. But most of all thinking it would be the last night my oldest child would sleep in our home as a single woman. Now she would have a different life, live in a new home and come home only for short visits.

When I woke up that morning, my lower jaw seemed to be moving from side to side. In other words, I had no control over it. Sometimes, only my right side would hit my top teeth upon closing my mouth, and other times it would only be my left side. Again, I blamed it on the stress and anxiety I was feeling that day. Fortunately, I did not let that ruin anything on that special day.

The following day, when everything was back to normal, I kept feeling the same thing. My doctor's office was closed for Christmas, so I could not do anything until he came back.

On January, 2002, I visited my doctor and explained what was happening. I even showed him, what I called my "unpredictable" jaw. The doctor seemed concerned, yet trying not to show it. He explained that the degeneration I had on my joint, especially the left one, was the cause of this.

This meant either I had to live with this problem or I would have to have a complete joint replacement of my left joint and a partial joint replacement of my right. The joints that would replace my joints would be artificial joints, which have a life expectancy of 3 to 10 years, depending on the patient.

At this time, I was not ready to deal with anymore surgeries, expecially one that from the start would not be permanent. So I decided on the first choice, I would learn to live with it.

For the next two months, I dealt with the pain and discomfort and the "unpredictable" jaw. The jaw exercises were not doing their magic anymore. The worse part was I was feeling more and more pain in my joint. As the pain was worsening, there were slight changes in my bite as well as the jaw structure. This could drive anyone insane, so I tried desperately not to give it much thought.

One day in school I'm teaching a class and felt my jaw was out of place. I kept opening and closing my mouth and felt the front teeth would not hit at all. I tried desperately to force my jaw into hitting the top and bottom front teeth, but nothing happened. When the class was over, I rushed to the bathroom, to look at myself in the mirror. What I saw was the same asymmetrical face I had, before the surgeries. In all honesty, I started to cry so much I could not find a way to get out of the bathroom. I had developed an open bite, the left side was plump, the right side was thinner and I had a protruded chin. I sat down on the toilet seat and started thinking of all I had gone through to end up this way. Even the pain was becoming intolerable as each day passed. I was back to where I started.

During those days, I had a monthly orthodontist appointment. I cancelled, because I did not want to face him or anyone for that sake. For my own good, I decided to reschedule. When the orthodontist saw me, he immediately told me I had to go see the doctor, which I affirmed. Yet I had no intention of going to see him.

Apparently, the orthodontist called my doctor, and his secretary called me to schedule and appointment. I accepted, but still had no intentions of going back to see him.

I felt I had no way out of this situation. When this doctor was recommended, I was told he was the best in my area. I had suddenly lost all faith in him. I wanted to find a better doctor and did not have the courage to tell him that.

After days of careful thought, I decided to go to the appointment. He was a very good doctor, who did exactly what he thought was best for me. He never lied about the risks involved in this surgery. I owed him, above everything else, honesty. He appeared very concerned about my well-being, and again suggested artificial joint replacement.

I would not have minded, if that would be the only option, but the fact that it was not a permanent solution, was in reality my main concern. I told him I was not happy with that option.

I left his office convinced there must be some other option better for me out there. I just had to start searching for more.

NINE

WHEN YOU SEARCH YOU FIND

I was starting to feel a state of depression I had never felt before. My TMJ was in my mind 24 hours a day. I could not sleep at night and just made it almost unbearable to go to work in the morning. I could not concentrate. My mind was in a constant blurr. People would talk to me and I was not even listening. All I was able to think of was TMJ.

I started, once again, feeling for my family. It was not fair to them. I would take care of them as a routine, but not the way I used to enjoy being in their lives. I would miss important meetings and doctor's appointment. You name it I felt it. And the feeling was not good.

This second time around, I was determined to search for answers. I searched the internet, went to the library to find books (to my surprise, very little is written on this subject) and talked to everyone I knew about it. I figured someone or something can shed light on this topic.

Then one day as I am talking to a co-worker, she mentioned a family member who had suffered a big fall and had damaged her TMJ. This person had been suffering for years and had gone through several surgeries with no relief. Then she went to a doctor who was doing an innovative surgery with less recovery time and had her surgery done.

She gave me the e-mail address of her relative, and I contacted her that same night.

As soon as I introduced myself, I explained my problem with TMJ. I proceeded to explain the surgeries and the consequences of these surgeries. I needed to find a permanent solution to this situation. She seemed to understand my feelings, as she had gone through a similar situation. She gave me the name, address and the telephone number of the doctor who had done the surgery. Her words as she gave me the information were, "he's expensive but the BEST!"

As I looked at the address, I realized this doctor was 4 to 5 hour driving distance from my house. This could definitely be a problem. Also, being expensive could also make it difficult for me, since we are hard-working middle class people.

When I turned my computer off that night, I had my mind going in circles. I decided not to mention any of this to my husband until the following day.

The following morning at school, I kept thinking of the word "expensive" and "distance". I didn't know if he accepted insurance. The surgery was a big one, which meant staying away from home for a long period of time.

I thought it was very idealistic to even think I could do this, but nontheless I decided to tell my husband.

That night at dinner, I told my husband the whole story. I even told him the way I felt about it, and how impossible I saw a way of going to this doctor. My husband immediately answered, "you don't know unless you try".

He was exactly right. How could I think this could be impossible, if I didn't give it a chance.

The following morning I asked for a half day at work so I could call the doctor's office long distance. At that point I wanted an appointment to see him, which the receptionist gave me a 2-day appointment for May 13-14, 2002. There was a fee for the two days and also a fee for an MRI I would have to have done during my visit. Also, 2-day stay in a near by hotel. This was in excess of $2,000.00.

The first appointment was on Monday, May 13 at 9:00 A.M. So I left my two youngest kids and our dog with my parents for those days and my husband and I set off at 4:00 in the morning to arrive there by the appointment time.

The waiting room was an elegant, yet simple place. There were two patients waiting to see him by the time we arrived. They were talking between them as we were waiting, and we heard them saying how much they had traveled to come see him. One was from Canada and the other from Virginia.

After hearing this I felt lucky, I'm only 4-5 hours driving distance.

My husband and I could not help but look at each other. We were both thinking similar thoughts; this was in reality the best doctor in this field or he could be the only one doing this kind of surgery. Whatever it was, I was starting to feel safe, and I was still in the waiting room.

My name was called and I follow the technician to a room. I laid down as she did a CAT Scan. Then she walked me back to the waiting room, where we picked up my husband and went into a room. Another person took panorex x-rays of my jaw area, and made a model of my mouth. Then she took me for some actual pictures of my face and teeth. Then we were taken to an office and I sat in a dental chair. There I would wait some time before anyone walked in. Finally, a very pleasant gentleman walked in. His appearance made me think he was the doctor. Yet he introduced himself as the assistant. He was a very qualified person, very knowledgeable and precise. He sat down next to me and started asking many questions. All my answers, he would write down on a piece of paper inside a folder. He started with my medical history ever since this all started, to which I answered very detailed in order not to miss anything important.

When I thought I had told him everything he needed to know, he asked me, "Have you ever received a blow to the head or jaw"? I had never been asked this question before that day and it seemed logical that I would say "No". I have never been punched or hit by anyone.

He noticed I had not understood the question, so he asked me if I had ever been involved in an accident. To this question I answered "yes". Now he wanted to know exactly what happened in this accident. It felt like an irrelevant question, since this accident had happened 11 years before. Still I explained the accident in detail. When I came to the part that I broke the windshield with my forehead, he asked me to stop. Now I knew what he meant by a blow to the head or jaw.

For the first time it dawned on me that my TMJ could have been caused by this accident.

Now that I knew the accident could have been a probable cause for my TMJ Disorder, I was full of questions.

What about the clenching of my jaw, which I had been doing unconsciously for years, and the soreness I felt on my jaw area years before this accident occured? I could tell he was the one asking, but the answers he would leave for the doctor. That was fine with me.

I had brought to this appointment, a copy of the MRI I had prior to the surgeries, copies of x-rays from the orthodontist, copies of x-rays and a file with more than 200 pages of report from my previous doctor. All these items he took and placed them on a small counter top facing a window with a gorgeous view of the bay. There was an empty chair in front of it, which I assumed was for the doctor. He excused himself for some time. The next person I would see would be the doctor.

An hour passed before the doctor walked in. He was a tall, well-mannered gentleman, which at first glance I realized he was someone I could trust. He introduced himself very courteously, and went straight to business.

He sat in the chair in front of the window, completely surrounded by x-rays and papers. He looked at all the x-rays and started reading each and everyone of the doctor's report. While he was concentrated in this, his assistant was reading aloud the information I had given to him in detail.

My husband and I looked at each other in astonishment. What kind of person could do all this at the same time? I figured, he's probably ignoring one or the other. Then to my surprise, he looked straight at me and asked me questions about what he had read and was being read to him.

After all this was finished, he examined me, while his assistant was measuring the length of my jaw on both sides, the width of my opening, etc...The doctor touched my joints for pain. I could only feel pain on the right joint, my left was almost painless. He asked me to have an MRI done that afternoon.

After leaving his office that afternoon, we had lunch and went straight to the MRI Center. I had the MRI done within an hour and we were free for the remainder of the day.

The following day we had our appointment at 2:00 P.M., which meant we could do anything we wanted in the morning. We decided to go for a swim in the hotel pool, then we had lunch and off we went to the doctor's office.

As soon as we arrived we were called in. This time, we were taken to a very small room with a round table and 4 chairs. We knew this was the talking room. In this room we would get all the answers we needed. A few minutes later, the technician walked in and placed a lap top computer on the table. She brought in the MRI results and placed them on the wall. She excused herself, and said the doctor would be in shortly.

The wait seemed endless, but finally the doctor walked in. He greeted us, and immediately sat in front of the computer. He told me to stand behind him to see what he was explaining as he brought up the screen. My husband also stood by me to see for himself. Through the computer, he was seeing the results of the CAT Scan I had taken the previous day. He measured the surface area of the right condyle, which was approximately 50% of normal standard, but the surface area of the left codyle measured less than 25% of normal standard. There had also been much more vertical degeneration on the left mandibular condyle.

In his opinion, a condyle in that degenerative state should be replaced, due to having a very high degree of risk of giving out.

He gave me two options for replacement; the artificial joint (which I already knew about and did not want) or bone grafting. His preferred option was bone grafting. As a matter of fact, he would not do an artificial joint replacement. In such case he would refer me to a doctor who would do it for me.

I wanted to know more about bone grafting. He would bone graft my own rib to rebuild the condyle. This piece of rib would be placed through two incisions on the left side of my face. The first is placed on the inside border of my ear, and the second is about a two inch incision along the lower jaw line. This graft would be protected by a fat graft surrounding the bone graft. This fat would be removed from my stomach by a small vertical incision under my belly button. The right condyle could still be saved by protecting it with a fat graft. Only one incision inside the border of the ear would be done. The latter one was to be taken into consideration after more careful review of the results from the MRI and the model done the previous day. With this type of reconstruction, it would be necessary to protect the healing tissues with braces, splint and heavy elastics for six to twelve months. I would have to stay in a near by hotel for approximately three weeks.

Now I was full of unanswered questions. What was the actual cause of my joint degeneration? His answer, though very obvious, caught me by surprise. The accident may not have been the actual cause, but could have aggravated an existing problem. It could have been the clenching of the jaw or any bad habits which caused this problem. And lastly, it could have been that I was born with weak jaw joints, and all the aforementioned could have worsened an already bad situation. Now that this question was answered, I had one more. Why does my right side hurt much more than my left if the left is the most degenerated one? The only explanation he could tell me was that due to the condition of the left condlye, the right was doing all the work, which was debilitating for an already sick joint.

In short, excluding the artificial joint replacement, the diagnosis and solution were as follows: The left joint was so degenerated it needed replacement with a rib graft. The right, which was also degenerated, but not as badly, could possibly be rebuilt using a fat graft.

In looking at my TMJ scenario, I would say, this was the best option I had heard thus far. In fact it could very well be my only option.

If I had this surgery, I would become part of a study, which has been done for years with very little percentage of failure.

It was two weeks before my 44th birthday. I had been suffering from TMJ Disorder for many years.

WOULD I BE WILLING TO SPEND THE REST OF MY LIFE SUFFERING FROM A DISORDER THAT WAS CHANGING EVERY ASPECT OF MY LIFE IN SUCH A NEGATIVE WAY?

Thinking about the rest of my life. I thought for an instant. I can not change the past, but I could sure change the future.

So my answer to this question was **NO!**

TEN

WHAT ABOUT THE COST?

After all was said and done, My husband being the money conscience person he is, asked for the price of this surgery. When I heard the cost would be about $50,000.00 my eyes opened in disbelief. I knew there was no way to come up with this kind of money.

I noticed that the cost issue was something that was not handled by the doctor, when he told us he had someone in the office who would be able to answer those questions for us, and this person was also in charge of scheduling surgeries. He asked his assistant to call him to the office. At this time, he wanted to make sure we had no other questions, then he courteously excused himself.

A few minutes later, a gentleman walked in. He greets us with a friendly smile. Honestly, he made us feel so comfortable, I was not shy about asking all sorts of questions about the cost of the surgery. Can they bill the insurance directly, before we pay? Does the doctor accept payments in installments? The answer to both questions was no.

He proceeded to explain on payment for the surgery. The total amount was to be paid the day before the surgery, preferrably through a Cashier Check. After the surgery, he will proceed to place the claim to my insurance, but in his years of experience he made us aware that the insurance company pays only a minimal amount for this surgery. The rest would come out of our pocket.

I had to ask the question. Where do people get this kind of money? My husband looked at me in astonishment.

He was in disbelief I would ask such a question. The answer to my question shocked me. He basically told me that when people are desperate they find the money. Boy, I did not expect to hear that, but it made sense.

After all my financial questions were answered, and none were what I wanted to hear, I was tempted to just say goodbye and go home. Instead I stayed, looked straight at him and asked, "Could my surgery be done in July?" He proceeded to open his scheduling book and answered, "July 24, 2002 at 8:00 A.M." I told him to put my name right there.

By the time we left his office that night, it was way past dinner time. We decided to go out to dinner and stay there that night. We would go back home on Wednesday morning. I could not believe what I had done. I had a surgery date and without the slightest idea of how we would pay for it.

I was ready to hear my husband ask me, "are you crazy?" Instead I heard those sweet and understanding words, "when we get back home, let's figure out how to pay for this so you can finally feel better". At this point, I felt so lucky to have someone who cared so much about the way I felt.

The four and a half hour trip back home felt like the longest trip I had ever taken. We were so quiet. It was hard to imagine, because my husband and I always find things to talk about. But this time we were both drowning in our thoughts. I bet he was thinking the same thing I was…MONEY!

For years, we had been paying off our mortgage. Every year we paid against the principal, and had already been mortgage free for eight years. Our plan had always been not to have mortgage payments so we could live a bit more comfortably. My husband is a truck driver and I have been a teacher for some years. Two professions which do not provide an opportunity for high income possibilities, so we figured that being debt free would help us live better. The last thing on my mind would have been to put a mortgage on our house.

When we got home, we spoke to my parents and aunt about the surgery and the cost. Immediately, they said they would help us out. At first, I felt uncomfortable, because the three of them are retired, and although they live somewhat comfortably, by no means do they have money to spare. Especially this kind of money.

I explained the total cost of everything, which was the surgery, three week stay in a near by hotel and six months without work after the surgery. Also, my husband would be staying with me during those three weeks, which meant he would not be working.

The following day, my family decided they would help with part of the surgery cost, the 3 week rental and some of the monthly expenses, while I was not working. I felt very grateful for all this, but felt it was not fair for me to take this kind of money from elderly people. I let them know I was not comfortable with that, but they insisted. When my family decides something, it is very hard to change their minds. Still, I realized they felt good helping us out and we needed all the help we could get.

I took out a piece of paper and started working with numbers. In total between the surgery, the hotel, the time without being able to work and some miscellaneous expenses, the amount would be in excess of $70,000.00. Finally, I knew how much I needed to come up with for the surgery. The next day I went to my bank and requested a small mortgage on the house.

Now that the money issue was resolved, I was ready to wait patiently for two months until the surgery date.

ELEVEN

PREPARING FOR THE SURGERY

I left my house on Wednesday, July 17. Exactly one week before the surgery. Since I was going to be away from home for so long, I wanted to take my family with me. This made me feel more secure. My two younger kids, my aunt and our dog left with us.

The day prior to leaving, I had my last appointment with the orthodontist. This time, to put the surgical wires and hooks. That appointment lasted approximately two hours, but this was a crucial part of the recovery after the surgery. The surgical wires can hold a great deal of pressure without breaking, and the hooks are the ones to hold the heavy elastics and the splint to keep my jaw closed.

I had reserved a villa close to the beach through the internet. It was about 15 minutes away from the doctor's office and the hospital, and a few minutes more away from the therapist. I wanted a place which allowed small pets, and close to the beach, so that my kids could enjoy a bit of their summer break. It did not turn out to be what we expected, but we decided to stay because of all the other conveniences.

On Friday, I had my first appointment. This time, I did not see the doctor. His assistant and technician were the ones who took care of me that day. During this visit, they made a splint, in order to simulate my corrected bite after the surgery. The splint would become part of my mouth for the next six to twelve months.

The assistant noticed the surgical hooks that the doctor likes to use were not the ones my orthodontist had placed. He then referred me to an orthodontist there who could put the right ones on within the same day. This was a $1,500.00 fee I was not counting with, but I had no choice but to do it anyway. These new hooks were a one-piece item with the surgical wires, so they were, indeed, much stronger. This could better withstand the pressure of the heavy elastics and the splint.

After this, we went to the hospital for the pre-op. We got back to the villa by 7:00 P.M. It had been a very long day, but we accomplished everything that day. This meant we had a free weekend. We tried to enjoy these days, prior to the surgery as if it were the last, at least for a long time.

On Saturday morning, my oldest daughter and her husband arrived. We went to the beach and had as much fun as possible. My son-in-law had to leave on Monday morning, but my daughter stayed for the surgery.

I did not have anymore appointments until Tuesday, July 23. This time my two daughters wanted to come along to meet the doctor.

When the doctor walked in, he asked how I was feeling. He wanted to know how nervous I was. In all honesty, I felt pretty calm. Only when I thought of how the actual surgery was going to be did I feel a bit anxious. He tried the splint that had been done on Friday. He tried it over and over and did not feel it was right. He asked the technician to correct what was wrong with it, but he still was not pleased. Finally, he took matters into his own hands and placed the model himself. Even the doctor had trouble making the splint, due to my bite. For a moment, there were five or six people in the small office, trying to help make the splint. For the first time, I started feeling a sense of anxiety. I even had thoughts of calling it quits. Suddenly, he said he had gotten the fit he was looking for. This fit is very important, because once the doctor fixes my bite during the surgery, the splint is the one who will prevent my bite from changing, until the joint heals.

Now that the model was perfect, the technician would have to make the splint. This would take about two hours.

By this time, it was already dark. The secretary gave me a beeper, and told me to go and eat somewhere close to the office so when it went off I could be there within 15 minutes.

We went to eat at a fairly nice restaurant across the street. I ordered a big salmon steak. I figured, I would eat healthy but alot, because this was going to be my last real meal for a very long time.

It was 9:00 P.M. when the beeper went off. I immediately headed for the office. The doctor tried the splint, and it fit perfectly. So we bid farewell, took all the prescriptions and headed to a pharmacy nearby. I took an Ativan before I went to bed that night. He told me not to have anything to eat or drink after midnight, but if I felt very anxious, I could take another Ativan when I woke up with very little water. Ativan was prescribed as an anti-spasmodic medication, but also relieves anxiety.

That night I slept like a baby. I really needed that sleep, because the following day I would face one of the hardest challenges of my life.

TWELVE

SURGERY NUMBER 4

I woke up that morning feeling very anxious. This surgery was the final hope for my TMJ Disorder. I took the Ativan to help me relax, just as the doctor had ordered. We got ready and I kissed my children goodbye. The next time I would see them would be after I would wake up from the surgery.

We arrived at the hospital at 6:00 A.M. The nurse took me in and asked me to change into the hospital robe. I put a head cap and a pair of surgical shoes. I put my clothes in a bag, which I gave to my husband to take to the room after the surgery. Then I laid in bed, waiting for another nurse to take me.

A few minutes passed and a nurse came in to take me to another room. The nurse prepared my I.V. By this time, I was getting extremely anxious. So many doubts came into my mind about the surgery. Though I knew this was my best choice, I also knew that anything could go wrong. Unfortunately, I knew from experience.

I asked her if she could put some calming medication, which she did, because all I can remember after that was the anesthesologist introducing himself. I know he explained the type of anesthesia he was going to sedate me with, but I do not remember a word he said. Now, I can only assume, he administered the same one I had on the previous surgeries.

I felt someone touch my face. It was the operating room nurse who was going to take me in to the operating room. She touched the part around my ears to show me where she was going to shave me for the surgery. I don't remember anything else after that.

I woke up at night and looked around the room. A nurse walked in and asked if I had any pain, which I could truly say I felt none. At that time I did not know what I had locking my jaw closed, but I could not open my mouth at all. I do recall noticing two small tubes, which connected from my face to a pocket I had on my robe. I took out a small rectangular piece, which looked like a beeper, from my pocket. The contents inside were blood. I soon realized, without looking at the mirror, I had two drainage tubes on each side of my face.

Not long after I woke up, my 3 kids walked in. They had been in the waiting room for hours. My younger daughter started turning pale and told me she was tired and had to go. I know her too well. She can not stand the sight of blood. My oldest daughter and my son stayed with me for a while, keeping me company. Then they left and my husband and aunt walked in and stayed a few minutes. They seemed very relieved that everything had gone so well.

By then, I was starting to feel pain, so the nurse showed me how to administer the morphine. I just had to press a button and the medicine would go through the I.V.

During the night, I was very itchy and had a terrible headache. It would not go away, not even after the nurse gave me a shot. I just turned the T.V. on to hear something. From my bed, I looked out a window, hoping I would see dawn.

Early that morning, my husband came in to see me. After he left the doctor and his assistant came in, and I explained the headache and the itching. He believed it could have been an allergic reaction to the morphine, so he changed the pain medication to Demerol.

Breakfast arrived while the doctor was there. All I could see were liquids. That was fine with me, because I was not hungry. I told the nurse I did not want anything, but the doctor insisted I drink something and walk around if I wanted to leave the hospital the following day. At lunchtime, the same thing came. I tried drinking a little, but I was full in no time. After lunch, the nurse took me for a walk around the hospital floor.

My husband was there most of the day, and also took me for short walks around. I felt very tired and dizzy, so I went back to bed.

I could not sleep very well that night. I just stayed up watching T.V. Everytime I felt some pain, I would press the button and the pain was gone. If everything would be that simple, life would be heaven.

The following morning the doctor and his assistant came, took out the drainage tubes and signed the discharge. After leaving the hospital, I went to his office to have a CAT Scan done.

After I left the doctor's office that day, I went straight to a church. I had to give thanks for all that had happened, and expecially the way I felt. I asked for a better future after this surgery, so I could be a better person and feel good about myself.

It was about 1:00 P.M. when we arrived at the villa. My parents had arrived that morning with tons of cooked food for us. My mom had made a soup, which she hoped I would eat. I took a few sips and went straight to bed.

I did not wake up until Saturday morning. When I woke up, I felt so good I even told my family to take me to the mall. I got dressed and we all left. As soon as I walked in the mall, people kept staring at me. I thought it was time to go, when I started feeling uncomfortable with the looks people were giving me.

For the first time since the surgery, I actually looked at myself in the mirror. I do not know what got into me, when I said I wanted to go to the mall, and my family not telling me anything. I was very swollen and had bruises around the ears. Still that did not give anyone the right to stare at me that way. I got to the villa and sat down to watch T.V.

During lunch, I had soup. I only took a few sips and went back to watching T.V. During that afternoon, I started feeling very weak, so I fell asleep for the rest of the afternoon. I woke up at dinner time to drink some soup and went back to sleep. I did not wake up until Sunday morning. All that day, I spent between bed and the sofa. I was not feeling much pain. The only pain I could feel was the rib area, other than that, the pain was very tolerable.

On Monday morning, I went to the doctor's office. I was already feeling so weak I could hardly walk. I just wanted to lie down and sleep. His assistant walked me to the office and sat me down in the dental chair. He offered some juice, but I could not drink it, because I also had a bad feeling in my stomach.

Before the doctor walked in, the assistant took off my elastics and the splint. The splint had been secured during the surgery with some wiring which he cut off at that time.

This was the first time in 5 days I felt free of that splint and elastics.

Soon after the doctor walked in and checked my opening. He gently put his fingers on my joint area. I was so happy to feel no pain for the first time in years. He looked inside my mouth and did some measurements. He walked us to a tiny room with a computer and explained the CAT Scan that was taken the previous Friday. He showed me the left condyle, which showed a piece of the rib attached with some screws. Then showed me the right condyle which showed the fat graft in place. I do not know much about it, but he was very pleased with what he saw. Everything was in place, and looking great after five days.

I then went back and sat in the dental chair, where the assistant taught me how to remove and place the splint and the elastics. I could take my splint and elastics off 5 times a day for 15 minute intervals. Every other week I would add 15 more minutes. During the time I had them off, I would eat, exercise with the therabite (this is a device that you place inside your mouth and forces your mouth to open as wide as you possibly can) and brush my teeth.

Before I left, the doctor asked about the pain from the surgery. All I could say was it was very tolerable. My only problem was the weakness and dizziness. Yet I knew as days went by it would slowly go away.

Immediately, I went to the therapist. I was feeling so weak, that upon laying me in a reclining chair and starting with a much relaxing heat therapy, I fell asleep. I was awaken by the therapist putting her hands on my face for some massage. This would go on every single day, except weekends, until I was discharged.

When I got to the villa that day, I made myself some spaghetti with meat sauce, then for dessert I pressed a banana with a fork and slowly ate it. I took all my medications and went straight to bed.

From that day on, I kept feeling better and better. My diet consisted of soft foods. I made it a point that if I could not press my meal with a fork, it was too hard for me to eat it.

The only problem I was having was with the Ativan. Although necessary for the spasms, it made me very sleepy. The doctor had prescribed it 4 times a day, but as soon as I explained, he told me to reduce it by half. This was a bit better, since I would take one when I woke up and the other one when I went to bed at night.

On Friday morning, I went to the doctor's office for suture removal. I was very nervous about that day, because I was full of stitches. On the left side of my face, I had stitches around my inner ear and a 2 inch stitched area close to my jawline. On my right side, I had stitches around my inner ear. To remove the piece of the rib, I was cut under my right breast, which left about 5 inches of stiched area there. Finally, my lower stomach had 2 inches of stitched area, where the fat was removed.

The assistant walked me into a room with a gorgeous view. I decided I would transport my mind into the bay area and pretend I was cruising in one of those beautiful sailboats, so I would not feel as every stitch is being pulled from my body. I was so mesmerized in the view, I hardly felt anything. Stitches had been removed from my stomach and under my breast. None were touched on my face. Those would ultimately fall out. I felt so relieved that when I left the office that day, I felt the worst had passed. From then on, I would focus on going back home.

We had a fairly nice weekend. I sat close to the pool with Amber on my lap, barking at everyone she saw. My husband and kids would be swimming and having fun in the pool and my aunt would sit inside watching T.V. My husband would cook BBQ and I would do some simple stuff for everyone to eat. I was starting to feel like my old self again.

On Tuesday morning, I visited the doctor in what would hopefully be, the last visit before going home. The doctor walked in right behind me and noticed how anxious I was to go home.

He examined all the wounds, asked me to open my mouth and measured the opening. It seemed I was already opening my jaw wider. He sat down and started talking to me about the feeling I had with the surgery. He was also concerned about the pain level I had felt due to the surgery and my joint area. I had no pain in my joint area, the pain in the surgery sights were almost none existent and I could truly say, I was very happy to have taken this step. Upon the completion of our conversation, he gave me the green light. I COULD GO HOME AT LAST! Those were the sweetest words I could ever hear. I would see him back in 6 weeks.

At home I would face some changes. I could not do everything I was used to doing, like answering the phone or cooking in front of the range for long periods of time. But other than that, I could do everything else.

For the past three weeks, we have been to the doctor's office several times, the hospital, the therapist, in short we had the works. Now it was time to head back to our quiet, loving home, one I now treasured more than ever.

THIRTEEN

A NEW BEGINNING

It's been six months since the surgery. I have no joint pain, the headaches are gone, I have more opening capacity (it is still not normal, but is getting there) and my face is slowly becoming symmetrical. The swelling on my left side will not completely improve until approximately a year. I'm still wearing the splint and the heavy elastics, but that is fine with me. I know this is what has made the recovery so great.

For so many years I have been feeling symptoms and discomforts from TMJ Disorder. For much of that time, I thought I would have to suffer with this for the rest of my life. I truly thought I had lost all faith in the cure.

Am I cured from TMJ Disorder?

I can not truly answer this question. I feel great right now. I am free of pain for the first time in years. I can look at myself in the mirror and feel good with what I see. Of course, I do not see a thirty-something woman anymore (which is when all this started), but I feel good about the way I look at forty-something.

I have learned so much from all these years. I have experienced many failures and successes. But through these experiences I have learned that giving up is not an option.

Crossing the bridge is sometimes very difficult. The bridge I had to cross was not an easy one. There were times, I thought of stopping in the middle or turn around and go back. Thanks to my determination and that of those people around me, I got the strength to keep going. With many obstacles on the way, I finally reached the other side. There I found exactly what I needed to get my life back. I wonder now, what would have happened if I had decided to stay half way, or worse turned around? I do not even want to think of that answer.

What actually caused my TMJ Disorder?

I will probably never know. It could have been the accident, the clenching of the jaw or simply I was born with weak jaw joint structure. I do know one thing for sure, the allergies and the acute colitis made the disorder more noticeable for me and triggered me to find a cure.

As time has gone by, I have realized that everything has a purpose. All this time, I wanted to be the way I was before all this started, instead I became a new and better person. **That's one thing I could thank my TMJ Disorder for.**

Yes, I am part of a study, and probably will be for the rest of my life. I just hope this could actually become the cure for all those people suffering from this disorder.

At this time, I do not know what the future will bring. I hope this will be my last surgery, but that I cannot foresee. I can only take care of myself as much as I can, and let nature take its course.

I admit my TM joints are in my mind every single day of my life. Now I think of them as my success story. One that could only be reached by always trying to see the light at the end of the tunnel.

No one ever said it was an easy crossing. Yet, in years to come, I hope I have taught my kids one very valuable lesson…**GIVING UP IS NEVER AN OPTION.**